HOMEMADE BEAUTY PRODUCTS

The Ultimete Recipe Collection of Homemade Deodorant, Homemade Soap, Homemade Shampoo, Homemade Body Butter, Homemade Cosmetics, Homemade Condiments And More!

BY

KATYA JOHANSSON

www.amazon.com/author/katyajohansson

« .Introduction. »

Natural Ingredients are the gifts of Mother Earth and are available in a wide variety of substances such as oils, butters, dried herbs or flowers, herbal powders, clays, salts, muds, essential oils, floral waters etc.

They can be used in simple or more complex recipes to make your own homemade natural hair and beauty products. Many natural cosmetic ingredients have superior therapeutic and skin/hair care properties in comparison to the synthetic ingredients often used in mass manufactured products. Manmade chemicals can also be toxic or harmful to health and are simply unappealing for those who have more natural lifestyle preferences.

Making your own natural products is also a fun, creative, relaxing and rewarding pastime. One which brings a sense of pride and nurturing both to yourself and loved ones when making products as gifts.

Table of Contents

1. Amazing Shea Butter Deodorant

Ingredients

- 3 T Coconut Oil
- 3 T Baking Soda
- 2 T Shea Butter
- 2 T Arrowroot (optional) or organic cornstarch
- Essential Oils (optional)

Method

1. Melt shea butter and coconut oil in a double boiler over medium heat until barely melted. Combine in a quart size glass mason jar with a lid instead and place this in a small saucepan of water until melted. This will save your bowl and you can just designate this jar for these type of projects and not even need to wash it out… This can also be done in the microwave if you have one.
2. Remove from heat and add baking soda and arrowroot (If you don't have arrowroot, use more baking soda or just omit)
3. Mix well
4. Add essential oils and pour into a glass container for storage. It does not need to be stored in the fridge.
5. If you prefer, you can let it cool completely and put into an old deodorant stick for easier use, though it may melt in the summer!

2. Best Coconut Oil Deodorant

Ingredients

- 6 T coconut oil
- 1/4 cup (4 T) baking soda
- 1/4 cup (4 T) arrowroot or organic cornstarch
- essential oils (optional)

Method

1. Mix baking soda and arrowroot together in a medium sized bowl.
2. Mash in coconut oil with a fork until well mixed.
3. Add oils if desired.
4. Store in small glass jar or old deodorant container for easy use.

3. Easy Natural Skin Care

Ingredients

- 2 tablespoons zinc oxide (Can use arrowroot powder instead if desired, but it will not offer quite as much coverage)
- 1 tablespoon arrowroot powder (optional)
- 1 teaspoon gold mica dust
- 1/2 – 1 tsp of desired natural clay powder (optional) I used a pinch of White cosmetic clay, Fuller's Earth Clay and French green clay
- up to 1 teaspoon finely ground cocoa powder OR bonze mica powder (or both) to get desired color
- Optional: 1 teaspoon of translucent mica powder can help for really oily skin

Method

1. Mix all ingredients to get desired color and coverage.
2. Zinc oxide will give coverage and matte finish.
3. Colored mica powders, natural clays and cocoa powder will give color. Start slowly and add as needed, testing on inner-arm as you go to find your shade.
4. Store in a small glass jar with a lid.

4. Wonderful Lotion Bars

Ingredients

- 1 cup coconut oil
- 1 cup shea butter, cocoa butter or mango butter (or a mix of all three)
- 1 cup beeswax
- Optional: 1 teaspoon Vitamin E oil

Method

1. Combine all ingredients (except essential oils if using) in a double boiler, or a glass bowl over a smaller saucepan with 1 inch of water in it. Combine in a quart size glass mason jar with a lid instead and place this in a small saucepan of water until melted. This will save your bowl and you can just designate this jar for these type of projects and not even need to wash it out...
2. Turn the burner on and bring water to a boil. Stir ingredients constantly until they are melted and smooth:
3. Remove from heat and add the essential oils.
4. Gently stir by hand until essential oils are incorporated.
5. Carefully pour into molds or whatever you will be allowing the lotion bars to harden in. I used these silicone baking cups, though any mold would work.
6. Allow the lotion bars to cool completely before attempting to pop out of molds. These could be made in different shaped molds for different holiday gifts or made in a square baking pan and then cut into actual bars.

5. Easy Homemade Lotion

Ingredients

- 1/2 cup Almond or olive oil
- 1/4 cup coconut oil
- 1/4 cup beeswax
- Optional: 1 teaspoon Vitamin E oil
- Optional: 2 tablespoon Shea Butter or Cocoa Butter
- Optional: Essential Oils, Vanilla Extract or other natural extracts to suit your preference

Method

1. Combine ingredients in a pint sized or larger glass jar. I have a mason jar that I keep just for making lotions and lotion bars, or you can even reuse a glass jar from pickles, olives or other foods.
2. Fill a medium saucepan with a couple inches of water and place over medium heat.
3. Put a lid on the jar loosely and place in the pan with the water.
4. As the water heats, the ingredients in the jar will start to melt. Shake or stir occasionally to incorporate. When all ingredients are completely melted, pour into whatever jar or tin you will use for storage. Small mason jars (8 ounce) are great for this. It will not pump well in a lotion pump!
5. Use as you would regular lotion. This has a longer shelf life than some homemade lotion recipes since all ingredients are already shelf stable and not water is added. Use within 6 months for best moisturizing benefits.

6. Best Homemade Sunscreen Bars

Ingredients

- 1 cup coconut oil (I get mine here)
- 1 cup shea butter, cocoa butter or mango butter (or a mix of all three equal to 1 cup)
- 1 cup beeswax (can add an extra ounce or two if you want a thicker consistency, which leaves less lotion on the skin when used)(I get mine here)
- 2 tablespoons (or more) of non-nano Zinc Oxide
- Optional: Vitamin E oil to preserve. I added 1 tsp vitamin E oil for this recipe made with 1 cup of each ingredient)
- Optional: a few drops of vanilla or essential oil for scent (do not use citrus oils!)

Method

1. Combine all ingredients (except zinc oxide and essential oils if using) in a double boiler, or a glass bowl over a smaller saucepan with 1 inch of water in it.
2. Turn the burner on and bring water to a boil. Stir ingredients constantly until they are melted and smooth:
3. Remove from heat and add the zinc oxide powder and essential oils.
4. Gently stir by hand until essential oils are incorporated.
5. Carefully pour into molds or whatever you will be allowing the lotion bars to harden in. I used these silicon baking cups, though any mold would work. This recipe exactly filled 12 silicon baking cups when I made it.
6. Allow the lotion bars to cool completely before attempting to pop out of molds. These could be made in different shaped molds for different holiday gifts (hearts for

valentines, flowers for Mother's day, etc.) or made in a square baking pan and then cut into actual bars.

7. They can be stored at room temperature or in the fridge or freezer for longer term storage. Keep below 80 degrees or they will melt! Adjust coverage to your needs and be careful not to burn while determining how long you can spend in the sun with these.

7. Amazing Dry Shampoo

Ingredients

- 1/4 cup arrowroot powder or organic cornstarch OR 2 tablespoons arrowroot/cornstarch + 2 Tablespoons cocoa powder
- 5 drops of essential oil of choice (optional- I use lavender)
- An old make-up brush to apply

Method

1. Put the drops of essential oil into the arrowroot or cornstarch and mix with a spoon. Store the mix in a small jar or old powder container.
2. Apply with an old make-up brush to the roots or oily parts of your hair. Applying with the brush is optional, but it removes the need to comb through as much and is better for styled hair. If you don't use the brush, comb the powder through your hair and style as usual.

8. Amazing DIY Wet/Dry Spray Shampoo

Ingredients

- 1 cup warm water
- 1/4 cup arrowroot or cornstarch
- 1/4 cup vodka, rubbing alcohol or witch hazel (what I use is from here)
- Essential oils or a spritz of your favorite perfume to scent

Method

1. Mix all ingredients in a small spray bottle and shake well. Shake before each use and spray on roots or oily parts of hair. Let dry and style as usual.

9. Amazing DIY Foaming Hand Soap

Ingredients

- 12-ounces of Water (distilled or boiled is best but not needed if it will be used within a few weeks)
- 2 Tablespoons Liquid Castille Soap (I get mine here at a discount)
- ½ tsp liquid oil like olive or almond
- Essential oils of choice for scent (optional)

Method

1. Fill the soap dispenser to about 1 inch of the top (leaving room for the bulky foaming pump and the soap to be added).
2. Add at least 2 tablespoons of liquid castille soap to the water mixture (NOTE: do not add the soap first or it will create bubbles when the water is added.
3. Add the oil (optional but it helps preserve the life of the dispenser) and any essential oils if you are using them.
4. Close and lightly swish to mix.
5. Use as you would any regular foaming soap.

10. Best Nourishing Hair Oil Recipe

Ingredients

- 2 Tablespoons olive oil
- 1 tablespoon coconut oil
- 1 tablespoon honey
- 1 teaspoon Epsom salt or magnesium flakes

Method

1. Combine all ingredients and whisk/blend well (I used an immersion blender). You may have to heat the coconut oil slightly to get it in liquid form. Epsom salt will still be somewhat gritty but will dissolve and work in to hair once applied.
2. Over a sink or shower, massage oil through the hair and scalp. Put a shower cap on (or old towel) and leave on for up to 30 minutes.
3. In the shower, rinse well, then shampoo. If still oily, massage a small amount of baking soda through the hair to remove or use dry shampoo after the shower.

11. Wonderful Shea Butter Soap

Ingredients

- 2 cups glycerin soap base, melted in a double boiler
- 2 tbsp shea butter, melted separately
- Several drops of your favorite essential oil (optional)

Method

1. Mix well, pour into molds (you can use regular food storage containers), and cool.

12. Amazing Whitening Sage Tooth Powder

Ingredients

- 1 tsp baking soda
- Table salt
- Dried sage

Method

1. Mix together 1 tsp each of baking soda, table salt, and dried sage.
2. Scoop onto a dampened toothbrush and brush as usual.

13. Amazing Body Butter

Ingredients

- 1/4 cup grated cocoa butter
- 1 tbsp coconut oil
- 2 tbsp sesame oil
- 1 tbsp avocado oil
- 1 tbsp grated beeswax

Method

1. Combine all the ingredients in an ovenproof glass container. Place the container with the mixture in a pan with a 1- to 2-inch water bath. Melt the oils and wax gently.
2. Pour the melted mixture into a clean jar and allow to cool. Stir the cooled mixture.
3. Spread the butter on your body and massage into the skin.

14. Basic Deodorant Powder

Ingredients

- 1/2 cup baking soda
- 1/2 cup cornstarch
- Antibacterial essential oils such as cinnamon, rose, birch or lavender, as preferred

Method

1. Place the baking soda and cornstarch in a glass jar. Add the essential oils; stir and cover.
2. Dampen a powder puff, cotton ball or sea sponge and dab into the mixture (or sprinkle the mixture on the sponge); pat underarms.

15. Best Homemade Deodorant

Ingredients

- Baking soda
- Cornstarch
- Anti-bacterial tea tree oil

Method

1. One of the best deodorants is plain old baking soda. You can pat it right onto your skin or mix it with a little cornstarch for extra staying power and moisture control.
2. Try ½ cornstarch and ½ baking soda. Some readers say that mixing in anti-bacterial tea tree oil makes it even more effective.

16. Homemade Easy Shampoo

Ingredients

- Castile soap
- Lemon juice
- 1 tsp salt
- ½ cup cornmeal

Method

1. Old-fashioned castile soap can also be dissolved in warm water to be used as shampoo.
2. After shampooing, rinse your hair with lemon juice to make it shine.
3. If regular shampooing with water is impossible for some reason, try mixing 1 tablespoon salt and ½ cup cornmeal in a shaker bottle. Sprinkle lightly onto hair, then brush thoroughly to get rid of dirt and oil. A combination of baby powder and cornstarch can also be used the same way.

17. Amazing Homemade Moisturizer

Ingredients

- Rosemary oil
- Castor oil

Method

1. For healthy skin, add rosemary oil to the bathwater.
2. Another age-old tradition to prevent wrinkles around the eyes is to apply a drop of castor oil around each eye before going to bed. Castor oil acts as a humectant, meaning that it attracts and retains moisture in the skin. This promotes healthier skin cell rejuvenation. Some plastic surgeons apply castor oil around an incision after surgery for this exact reason.

18. Easy Eye Make-up Remover

Ingredients

- 1 tsp canola oil
- 1 tsp castor oil
- 1 tsp olive oil

Method

1. Save on those very expensive eye make-up removers with this recipe. Combine 1 tablespoon canola oil, 1 tablespoon castor oil, and 1 tablespoon light olive oil.
2. For use on your entire body, put some castor oil in a little spray bottle. To maximize absorption, spray it on your skin after showering and gently rub it in while your skin is still warm and your pores are open.

19. Amazing Natural Skin Cleanser

Ingredients

- Fresh milk or butter milk
- Lavender oil

Method

1. As the tub fills, pour in two cups to one quart of fresh milk or butter milk. Fresh milk can be substituted with one cup of powdered milk. A few drops of lavender essential oil may increase the relaxing effects.
2. Soak in the tub for at least 20 minutes and gently massage your skin with a wash cloth or a loofah to rub off all the dead skin.
3. After taking your bath, drain the tub and take a quick shower to rinse off all the milk on your body.

20. Wonderful Oatmeal Soap

Ingredients

- ½ cup oatmeal, ½ cup small soap pieces
- 1 and ½ tablespoons cooking oil
- 1 tablespoon water

Method

1. If you have leftover soap slivers in the bathtub or sink, you can recycle them into this yummy new soap! Oatmeal has proven moisturizing benefits.
2. Gather these ingredients: Put the soap slivers in a plastic bag and pound them into small chunks.
3. Put chunks in a blender, add the oatmeal and pulse until grainy.
4. Pour into a bowl and add the oil and water.
5. Mix with your hands, removing any remaining bigger chunks of soap.
6. Shape the mixture into a ball and let sit until hard, about two hours.
7. Be sure to wash the blender thoroughly to remove the soap residue.

21.Homemade Best Deodorant

Ingredients

- 2 tbsp. beeswax granules
- 1¼ tbsp. shea margarine, cocoa
- 2 tbsp. beeswax granules
- 1¼ tbsp. shea margarine, cocoa spread, mango margarine, and so on.
- 1¼ tbsp. coconut oil
- ½ tbsp. bentonite earth

Method

1. In a twofold heater, or a little pot over low warmth, join the beeswax, coconut oil, and shea margarine until liquefied totally and blended well. 2. Expel blend from warmth and empty fluid into a glass or plastic packet or container.
2. Expel blend from warmth and empty fluid into a glass or plastic compartment. Rush in the heating pop (or arrowroot) and bentonite earth until all around consolidated. Note: You need to ensure the bentonite earth does not touch any metal, as it can adversely ...
3. Expel from warmth and let cool for a couple of minutes and after that mix in your vital oils. ...
4. Take an old (clean) antiperspirant stick and ensure the plunger thing is contorted the distance down. Deliberately empty your warm blend into the compartment.
5. Let sit with the top off until it has cooled totally. At that point, use as ordinary.

22. Homemade Deodorant

Ingredients

- 4oz+ jar or tin
- Double-boiler
- Kitchen scale
- 30g Coconut oil
- 20g Shea butter
- 10g Carrier Oil
- 10g Beeswax
- 15g Arrowroot powder
- 15g Diatomaceous Earth
- 5 drops of Vitamin E
- 20-25 drops of essential oils

Method

1. Measure oils, shea butter, and beeswax into the upper part of your double-boiler (for me, this is a glass bowl)
2. Melt on low heat over bottom part of double-boiler (for me, a pot with shallow water) until everything is melted (the beeswax will be the last thing to melt...just keep stirring)
3. Turn off heat and allow to cool for a few minutes
4. Add arrowroot, DE, Vit E, and EO; whisk vigorously to fully combine
5. Pour into container and place somewhere safe so it can set up (which actually doesn't take very long)

23. Amazing Natural Deodorant Ever

Ingredients

- 1 lemon

Method

1. Wash a lemon.
2. Cut lemon in half.
3. Squeeze a small amount of juice into your hand.
4. Rub onto armpits.

24. Wonderful Homemade Deodorant

Ingredients

- 4 tsp arrowroot powder
- 3 tsp shea butter
- 2 tsp coconut oil
- tsp baking soda
- 1/4 tsp essential oil of your choice

Method

1. Melt the coconut oil and shea butter over low heat until melted.
2. Combine the remainder of the ingredients.
3. Mix well and let cool.
4. Store in a small jar like these jars.
5. Apply as often as you'd like- (I apply once in the morning)

25. Non-toxic Citrus Easy Deodorant

Ingredients

- 6 tsp coconut oil, melted
- 1/4 cup baking soda
- 1/4 cup arrowroot powder
- 15-20 drops lemon essential oil

Method

1. Combine baking soda and arrowroot powder in a bowl and mix with a fork
2. Mash in the coconut oil until a nice paste forms
3. Add in essential oil to your scent level preference
4. Scoop into jar
5. I used these jelly jars for mine because they are so cute!
6. Use Non-toxic Citrus Homemade Deodorant as needed. The smell is very refreshing and I can honestly say that I have never had a better working deodorant!

26. Vanilla Bean Body Butter

Ingredients

- 1 container crude cocoa margarine
- 1/2 container sweet almond oil
- 1/2 container coconut oil
- 1 vanilla bean

Method

1. Melt cocoa spread and coconut oil. Expel from warmth and let cool for 30 minutes.
2. Grind a vanilla bean in an espresso processor on the off chance that you have one. If not, utilize a nourishment processor.
3. Blend sweet almond oil and vanilla bean bits into the cocoa spread and coconut oil.
4. Place in cooler to chill – around 20 minutes. Hold up until oils begin to somewhat harden.
5. Whip with an electric blender or in the sustenance processor until a spread like consistency is accomplished.
6. Spoon into a glass jolt and appreciate! Makes approximately 3 glasses whipped spread – keep in the fridge or another cool spot.

27. Amazing Rosemary Hair Oil

Ingredients

- 1 C Olive Oil
- 1 C Coconut Oil
- ½ C Rosemary Leaves
- ½ C Nettle Leaves
- ½ C Calendula Flowers

Method

1. Put the herbs into a glass mason jar or a medium sized Pyrex measuring bowl and cover with the oils. Place the glass jar or bowl into a pot of water, using the "double boiler method" and turn the pot of water on medium low.
2. This applies heat to the oils and herbs and allows them to infuse without getting too hot. Allow the herbs and oils to infuse for 4-6 hours, mixing occasionally. Strain out the herbs, squeezing out all the essential volatile oils, and store your oil in a clean, dry, lidded glass jar.

28. Easy Rosemary Herbal Shampoo

Ingredients

- 1 C Dr. Bronner's Liquid Castile Soap – Unscented (I get mine here)
- 1 C Glycerin (I get mine here)
- 1 Tbsp Oil. You can use the rosemary hair oil, almond, jojoba, fractionated coconut, or olive.
- 15-20 drops of Rosemary Essential Oil

Method

1. Combine the ingredients in a bottle and shake vigorously before each use. Use as you normally would in the shower.
2. The glycerin in the shampoo is there to add a nice foamy feel, like you would get from a normal shampoo. If you don't mind not having that foamy feel, you can use water instead.
3. Some people prefer less castile soap, as it can leave hair feeling oily. In this case experiment cutting the amount of soap and replacing it with water until you find the ratio that works best for you.

29. Amazing Rosemary Hair Rinse

Ingredients

- 1 C Boiling water
- 1 Tbsp Rosemary leaf, fresh or dried

Method

1. Pour the boiling water over the rosemary leaves, cover, and let it steep for 10-15 minutes. Strain out the herbs. Let it cool to warm, but not hot, while still covered. Once the water is a suitable temperature hold your head over a bowl and pour the rosemary infusion over your hair.
2. Take the water from the bowl, pour it back in a glass, and pour it over your hair again. Keep doing that until there is no more rosemary infusion left. This is best done right after a shower when your hair is already wet.

30. Easy Rosemary Vinegar Hair Rinse

Ingredients

- ½ C Rosemary leaves
- ½ C Nettle leaf
- ½ C Peppermint leaf
- 15-20 drops Rosemary Essential Oil
- 2 C Raw Apple Cider Vinegar

Method

1. Place the dried herbs in a sterile glass jar and cover with apple cider vinegar. Top off after a day or two after the herbs absorb some of the ACV.
2. Shake the jar daily for two weeks and allow the herbs to infuse into the vinegar.
3. After two weeks strain the herbs from the vinegar and store it in a lidded glass jar, out of direct sun light.

31. Homemade Shampoo

Ingredients

- 1 C Dr. Bonner's Liquid Castille Soap
- 1 C Glycerin
- 1 Tbsp Almond or Jojoba oil
- 15-20 drops of Essential Oils

Method

1. Combine ingredients in a recycled shampoo bottle, shake well, and use like any other shampoo.
2. This shampoo is fine to be stored in the shower and is good for a year.

32. DIY Natural Dry Shampoo

Ingredients

- 1/2 cup arrowroot powder
- 1 tablespoon cocoa powder (adjust according to hair color)
- A clearly awesome individual with slightly greasy hair

Method

1. Mix. Apply small amounts. Comb and tussle hair. Continue being awesome

33. Easy Body Butter

Ingredients

- 1 cup organic raw shea butter (solid)
- 1/2 cup coconut oil (solid)
- 1/2 cup almond oil (liquid)

Method

1. Melt shea butter and coconut oil in the top of a double boiler. Remove from heat and let cool for 30 minutes.
2. Stir in almond oil and essential oils of your choice. Place oil mixture in freezer or outside to chill.
3. Wait until oils start to partially solidify then whip until a butter-like consistency is achieved. Place in clean, glass jar and enjoy! A little goes a long way.

34. Lavender Superb Body Butter

Ingredients

- 4 Tbsp Coconut oil
- Tbsp Olive oil
- 2 Tbsp. Beeswax
- 1 Tsp. Honey
- 3 Tbsp. Aloe Vera gel
- 2 Tsp. Lanolin
- 10 drops Lavender essential oil
- 1 Vitamin E capsule

Method

1. In double boiler over medium-high, heat oils, beeswax and honey.
2. In a separate double boiler over medium-high, heat aloe. Once melted, mix into beeswax mixture. Stir.
3. Add lanolin & stir.
4. Once mixture has melted, turn heat to low. Stir in Vitamin E and essential oil. Whip until smooth.
5. Pour into small glass jars and let cool before covering.

35. Amazing Body Butter

Ingredients

- 1 cup coconut oil
- 1 teaspoon vitamin E oil (optional)
- a few drops of your favorite essential oils for

Method

1. Put all ingredients into a mixing bowl. Do not melt the coconut oil first. It will only whip up if it's solid.
2. Mix on high speed with a wire whisk for 6-7 minutes or until whipped into a light, airy consistency.
3. Spoon the whipped coconut oil body butter into a glass jar and cover tightly. Store at room temperature, or in the refrigerator if your house is so warm it melts the oil.